Weeb Ewbank's

PRO FOOTBALL WAY
TO
PHYSICAL FITNESS

by WEEB EWBANK
Head coach of The New York Jets
and

LUD DUROSKA

GROSSET & DUNLAP
A NATIONAL GENERAL COMPANY
Publishers · New York

A Castle Books, Inc. Edition
Distributed To The Trade
By Book Sales, Inc.

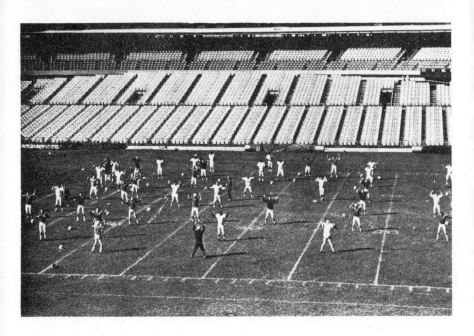

Photographs by Bart Silverman

Contents

1

The Need for a Physical Fitness Program

Thanks to the marvelous technological age in which we live—the age of automation, television and household conveniences—Americans probably have never been in poorer physical condition.

The evidence is sobering. According to one national survey, more than half of the children in the fourth to eighth grades failed to average sufficient daily exercise to properly develop their growing bodies.

In tests conducted by the President's Council on Physical Fitness, a third of the students failed to measure up to even minimum fitness standards. Another survey showed that the average teen-ager watches television from 15 to 30 hours a week and devotes only two hours to exercise and sport.

Many adults are in a similar sad state. Sedentary jobs are a prime cause of heart disease. Men who physically exert themselves at work suffer half as many heart attacks as a comparable group of desk-sitters and button-pushers.

The fitness problems of "white-collar" men are so commonly recognized that at a national conference on cardiovascular diseases, the recommendation was made that office-workers receive a 10-minute break every day to exercise!

The average man is fully grown at the age of 25 and, if he is fit then, his weight should not greatly increase in later life. But how many can say they have held the weight line?

What about the man who participates regularly in a recreational sport? Does he have to be concerned about his physical condition? The answer is yes. While engaging in a sport is a useful and pleasurable complement to a fitness program, it is by no means the whole solution. The same muscles tend to be used over and over again, and the others are neglected.

The remedy, most medical authorities agree, is a program of regular and planned exercise that involves the entire body. Coupled with intelligent eating, sleeping and working habits, a well-organized conditioning program enables you to achieve the prize of physical fitness.

Even professional athletes require consistent, year-round attention to exercise. Coaches have long realized that the closer to top condition the players are in when they report to training camp, the more quickly they reach their maximum potential.

Obviously it is not our intention to build you into pro football players. Even though the pro is well above average in strength and physique, we have learned with the Jets that he needs a regular physical conditioning program. What applies to him in some measure applies to you. The exercises—the calisthenics, isometrics and weight-lifting—that have been tested and recommended for the Jets' players offer a safe and sound method, when properly used, for you to improve your health.

The special section on stretching exercises can be of help to everyone regardless of age. Devised by Dr. James Nicholas, the Jets' team physician and an orthopedic surgeon, the exercises are especially valuable in cases where more flexibility of the joints and muscles is needed.

The extent of your personal conditioning program depends, naturally, on many things, including your age, your general state of health and your physical goals. Everyone's needs vary, and you should consult your doctor before undertaking a vigorous program. The schedules listed throughout the book are not meant to be rigid but rather to serve as a guide. Use common sense in modifying them to your requirements.

Your diligence in carrying out a sound conditioning program should be well-rewarded. By making your heart and body function more efficiently, you will derive many benefits. It will help you to be a better student or worker, improve your appearance, bolster your self-confidence and, happiest thought of all, perhaps enable you to live longer.

2

Test for Fitness

Here's an easy test which anyone can take at any age to find out how well his circulatory system is functioning and, in general, how fit he is.

When relaxed and rested, take your pulse (place two fingers of one hand against the inside of the wrist of the other hand and count your pulse beat for 30 seconds). Then double the figure to obtain your normal pulse rate. The figure itself is not significant since pulse rates vary among individuals regardless of their physical condition. What is important is how much of a change occurs in the pulse rate after the test.

Stand upright and assume a runner's position. Run in place, lifting your legs at least six inches off the ground, at a quick tempo. Count each time your foot touches the floor until you reach 100 or if more convenient, count each time your left foot touches the floor until you reach 50. Take your pulse. Then rest for two minutes and take your pulse again. The margin of difference from your normal pulse rate will provide a clue as to how much exercising you will have to do to achieve an adequate level of fitness.

If your pulse rate immediately after the test has doubled from the normal rate, say to 160 or more, and then has not slowed greatly after the two-minute rest, you should see your doctor for a physical examination.

As you exercise regularly, the margin between the "before and after" pulse rates should grow smaller. When the two rates are the same or within a count or two, then your general physical condition is good. Your normal pulse rate also should decrease.

3

Calisthenics for the Young Man (Ages 13 to 25)

A sound physical conditioning program starts with calisthenics and *always* includes calisthenics. They tone up and firm all the major muscles of the body and strengthen the circulatory system, making the heart and lungs work more efficiently. They help in maintaining strength, agility and endurance. Regardless of how high a level of fitness you achieve, you should never think you have advanced beyond calisthenics. Don't discard them for isometrics and/or weight-lifting. Even the best-trained athletes continue to do calisthenics as an essential part of their workouts.

This calisthenics program is intended to supplement whatever exercising you may do at school or at work, unless you are already training intensively as a member of a sports team.

The most direct route to physical self-improvement is to perform the exercises regularly. Try to maintain a five-days-a-week schedule with Saturday set aside for the weekly run-walk exercise. It will be helpful if you can exercise at about the same time each day so that it becomes a normal part of your routine.

It is important to do each exercise properly. So read the descriptions under the photographs carefully. At the beginning, be more concerned with performing each exercise thoroughly rather than with how fast you can finish. You are not competing with anyone else—only with yourself.

How much rest you will need between exercises will depend, naturally, on your condition. This program was planned to begin with a minimum level of physical activity. If you have been "checked out" by your doctor, you should be able to complete the minimum number of repetitions with few "breathers." However, rest at any time when you become too fatigued or if you feel pain. Your muscles may be a little sore or stiff the next day at the start, but you should not have any serious discomfort. As you progress, you will find you will need fewer "time-outs" until you are able to do the whole set without any pauses.

The sequence of calisthenics and the number of repetitions are suggested guidelines. It would be helpful to talk to your physical education teacher, coach or doctor about which of the calisthenic exercises would prove more beneficial according to your individual needs.

Basic Level Schedule

		Repetitions	
		Mini-mum	Maxi-mum
Page No.	Exercise	mum	mum
10	Jumping Jacks	10	20
9	Arm Circles (each way)	20	30
11	Side Twisters	10	20
12	Toe Touching	10	20
13	Sit-Ups	10	15
14	Push-Ups°	5	10
15	Running in Place	100 counts	
15	Weekly Run-Walk	¼ to ½ mile jogging *or* 4 50-yard runs alternated with 50-yard walks	

° Push-ups will probably be the most difficult exercise. If they are too hard to do at the beginning, substitute knee push-ups but return to the regular push-ups as soon as you build sufficient strength in your arms and shoulders.

Start with the minimum number of repetitions. Complete the entire set in five minutes before increasing the repetitions to the maximum. Again, the goal should be to complete the exercises in five minutes. After you succeed for five straight days, you are ready for the Medium Level.

Note: The daily workout may be skipped on any day in which you compete in a sport, provided it is reasonably strenuous.

BASIC LEVEL

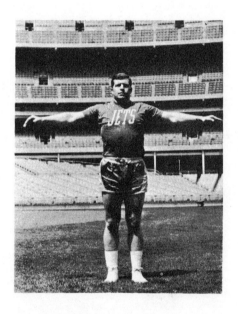

Arm Circles: Extend arms directly out to the side at shoulder height with palms down, fingers straight and together. Rotate the shoulders in forward motion so that the arms describe circles of about a foot in diameter. At the same time arch the head backward and turn it slowly to the left and to the right. After completing the specified number of repetitions, rotate the shoulders in a backward motion for the same number of repetitions. Be sure to keep the arms straight and do not let them "droop."

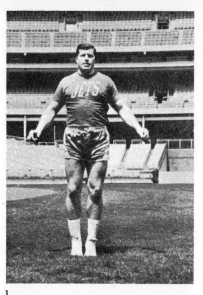

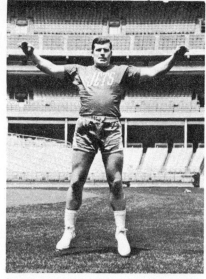

1

2

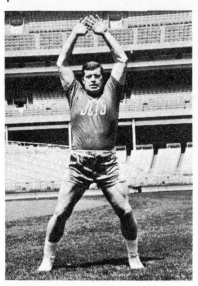

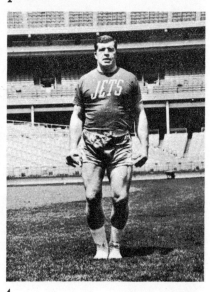

3

4

Jumping Jacks: Assume an at-attention position, with shoulders back, chest out, stomach in and arms straight down. Swing your arms in a full arc over your head until your fingers touch and simultaneously jump so that your feet land about shoulder-width apart. Hold for an instant and jump back to starting position. Hold for an instant and repeat. The exercise should be done in an almost continuous, rhythmic motion.

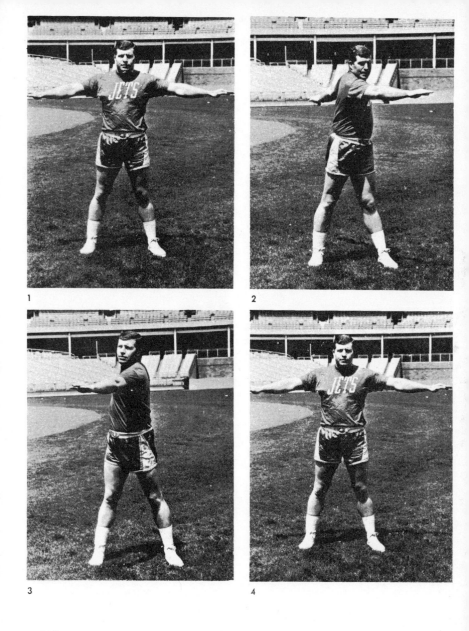

1

2

3

4

Side Twisters: Place feet shoulder-width apart and arms extended straight to the side at shoulder-level. Keeping feet stationary, twist trunk to the left as far as you can and return to starting position. Then twist to the right as far as you can and return. Keep arms straight and do not let them drop.

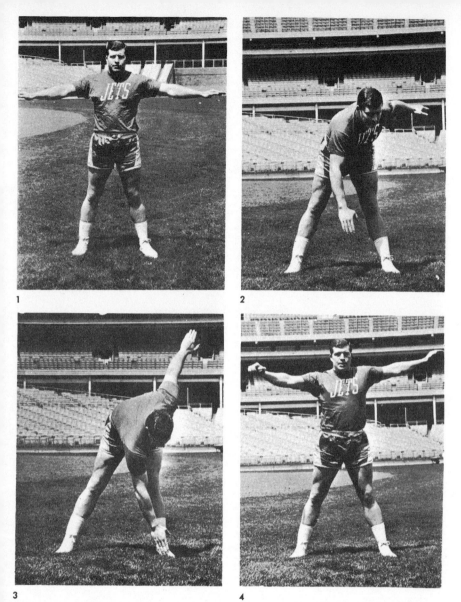

1

2

3

4

Toe Touches: Place feet shoulder-width apart and arms extended to the side at shoulder-level. Bending from waist, try to touch right foot—or as close as you can—with left hand, keeping knees straight. Return to starting position and repeat with right hand to left foot. Avoid strain to lower back and calves.

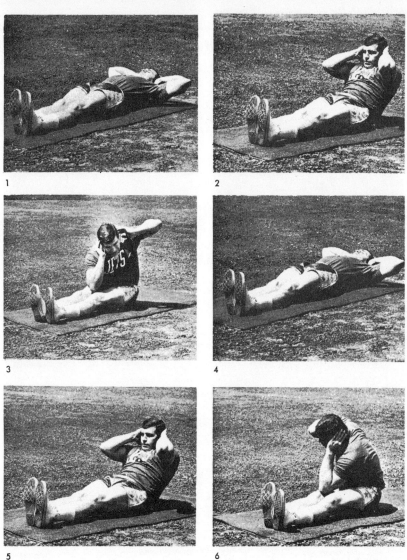

Sit-Ups: In the photographs, the Jet player is performing a more difficult version of the sit-up. It is better to start with the easier one, and then progress to the harder. Stretch out on the floor on your back with arms over your head and legs together. Contracting your stomach muscles, bring body up and touch toes. Keep legs straight. Return to starting position. If you have a problem raising yourself, put your feet under a heavy object—such as a sofa or desk—to anchor them. (NOTE: On Medium Level and Advanced Level, perform exercise as illustrated.)

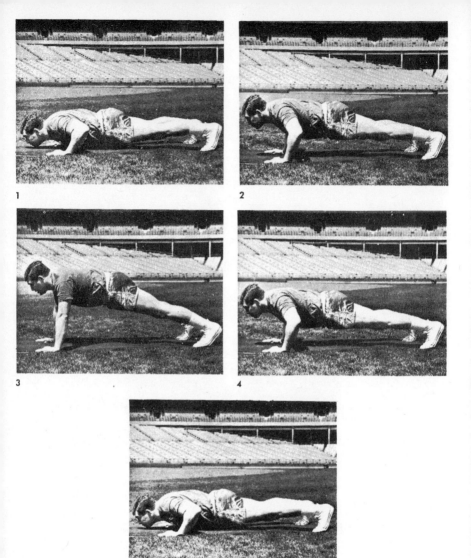

Regular Push-Ups: Stretch out on the floor on your stomach, with your hands underneath your shoulders, fingers forward. Push on your hands and raise yourself until your arms are straight and your body is resting on your hands and toes. Hold for a second and lower your body until it nearly touches the floor. Then raise yourself again. Don't let back sag—it should be straight—and don't push buttocks up first. The arms should do the work.

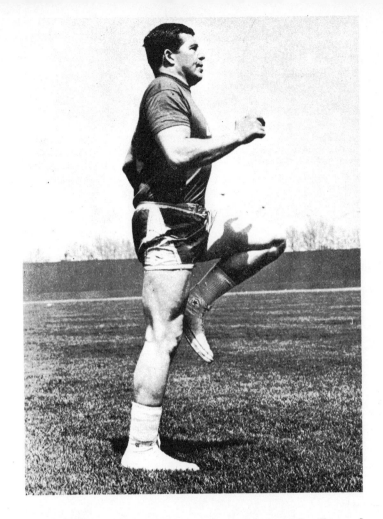

Running in place: Assume runner's position with elbows bent. Keep shoulders back and body straight. Lift legs at least six inches off floor. Count each time left foot hits floor. Start slowly and then speed up.

WEEKLY RUN-WALK EXERCISE

Since individual capacity varies so greatly, you should adapt this exercise to your needs and purposes.

For general conditioning, jog about a quarter of a mile (about 2½ city blocks). If you become winded, slow down to a walk until you feel able to resume jogging. In a few weeks you should jog the entire way comfortably. A satisfactory substitute would be any sport that requires running. The run-walk exercise can also be replaced by swimming the same distance, using any stroke.

If your goal is to develop speed, run at moderate or three-quarters speed for about 50 yards. Then walk about 50 yards. Repeat three times, running as fast as you can each time.

Medium Level Schedule

		Repetitions	
		Mini-mum	Maxi-mum
Page No.	Exercise		
10	Jumping Jacks	20	30
9	Arm Circles* (each way)	30	30
11	Side Twisters	20	30
12	Toe Touches	20	30
24	High Kicks (each leg)	5	10
17	On All Fours	4	8
13	Sit-Ups**	10	15
19	Knee to Chest (each knee)	10	15
14	Push-Ups	10	20
18	Leg Crossovers	4	8
15	Running in Place	200 counts	
15	Weekly Run-Walk	½ to 1 mile jogging *or* 6 50-yard runs alternated with 50-yard walks	

* Hold a book or small weight in each hand for a more effective exercise.
** Perform exercise as illustrated.

Be your own pace-setter. Increase the number of repetitions gradually, at first with those exercises you find easiest. Time is not a factor here. It is more important to do all the exercises vigorously. Your goal should be to complete the schedule without a "breather." After achieving this goal for five straight days, you can proceed to the Advanced Level.

Take the Fitness Test and note the changes in the pulse rate.

MEDIUM LEVEL

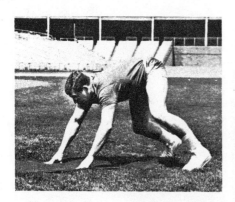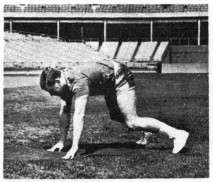

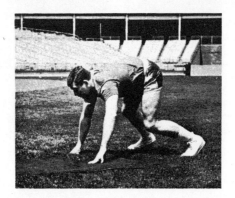

On All Fours: Bend down and place your hands, fingers forward, about 12 to 18 inches in front of your feet. Hop to the left, then forward, then to the right and then backward to the starting point.

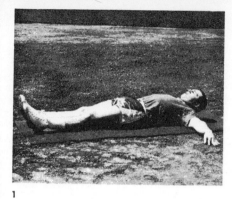

1

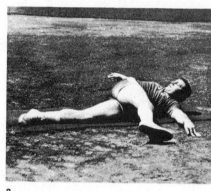

2

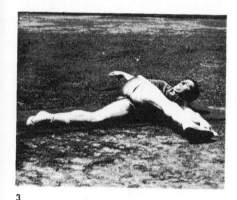

3

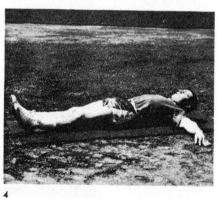

4

Leg Crossover: Stretch out with legs together and arms extended to the side. Lift right leg and cross over, twisting from the waist, and try to touch left hand with right foot. Return to starting position and repeat with other leg. Try to keep both legs straight.

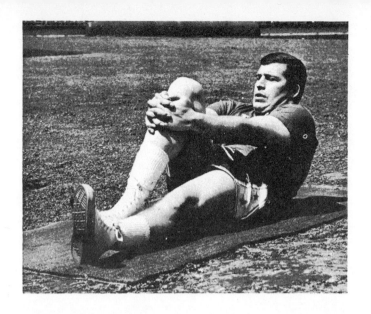

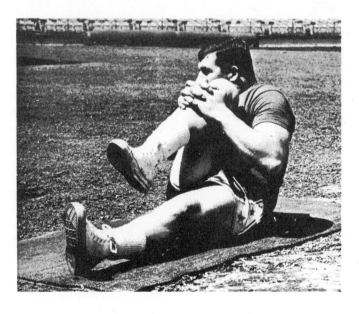

Knee to Chest: Sit with legs straight. Bring your right knee up, clasp your hands around the shin and pump the knee vigorously to chest. Return to starting position. Repeat with left knee.

Take the Fitness Test and note the changes in the pulse rate.

Advanced Level Schedule

Page No.	Exercise	Repetitions Minimum	Maximum
10	Jumping Jacks	30	40
9	Arm Circles	30	40
11	Side Twisters	30	40
	or		
21	Trunk Twisters*	15	30
12	Toe Touches	30	40
24	High Kicks (each leg)	10	10
17	On All Fours	8	12
22	Leg Lifts	10	20
13	Sit-Ups	20	30
	or		
23	Abdominal Curls*	10	20
14	Push-Ups	20	30
18	Leg Crossovers	8	12
25	Chin-Ups	5	10
15	Running in Place	300 counts	
15	Weekly Run-Walk	1 to 2 miles jogging	

* Use this alternate exercise as you find yourself mastering the schedule.

Concentrate on those exercises that prove hardest to do properly with the required number of repetitions.

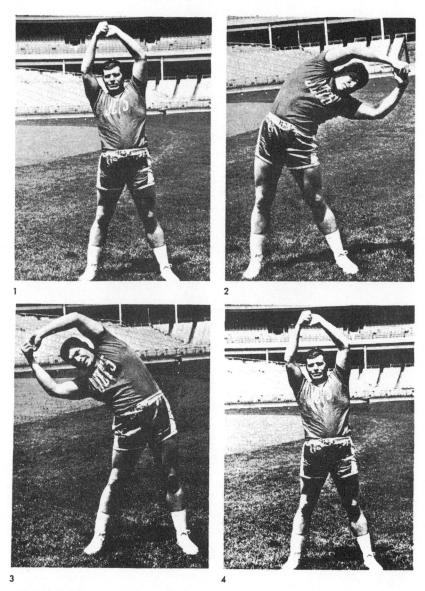

Trunk Twister: Place feet shoulder-width apart with arms overhead and hands clasped in reverse grip. Lean from waist to the left as far as you can, then forward, then to the right and then backward, rotating the upper part of the body in as big a circle as possible. Keep the feet stationary and arms straight.

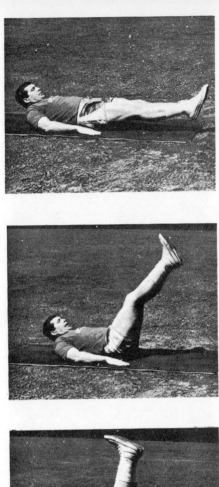

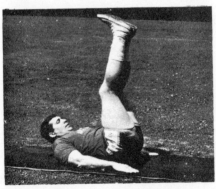

Leg Lift: Lie on your back with arms down at your sides and legs straight and together. Raise your legs as high as you can. Use your arms only to keep your balance—not to help bring your legs up.

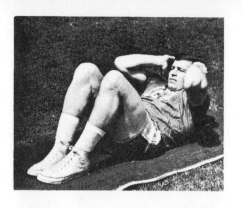

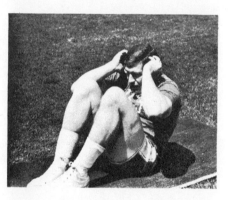

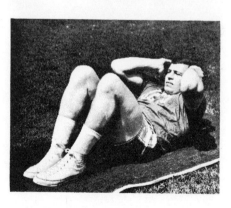

Abdominal Curl: Lie on your back with hands clasped behind head, knees bent and feet flat on the floor. Contracting stomach muscles, bring body up and touch elbows to knees and return to starting position. Try to keep feet flat on ground. Use the abdominal muscles and not the upper part of the body.

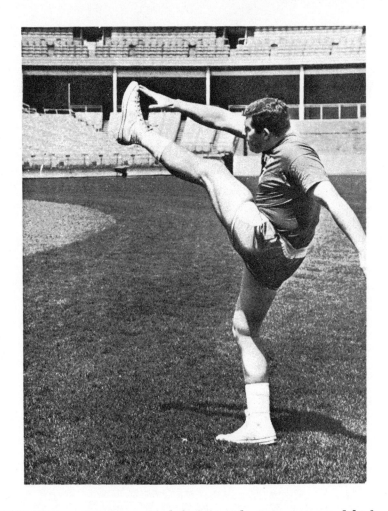

High Kick: Starting with left foot, take two steps and kick as high as you can with left leg. Step back to starting position. Take two steps, starting with right foot, and kick as high as you can with right leg. Quicken tempo, but avoid undue strain on calves.

Chart your progress by taking the Fitness Test again.

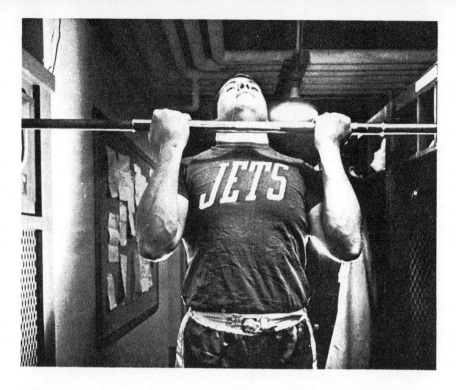

Chin-Ups: The bar should ideally be high enough so that you can "hang" by your hands from the bar without your feet touching the floor. If the bar is lower, bend the knees to avoid touching the floor. Grasp the bar with your palms toward you, shoulder-width apart. Pull yourself up until your chin is slightly above the bar. Then lower to starting position. Rely on your arms and shoulders to do the pulling. Do not let the body sway, and avoid "kicking" on your way up.

Congratulations! Being able to complete this schedule without difficulty puts you far above the average in physical condition. Once you have reached the peak, you should continue to do the exercises daily or at least every other day to maintain your fitness. The schedule also may be modified if you include any stretching, isometric or weight-lifting exercises.

4

Calisthenics for the Varsity Athlete

These exercises, since they stress the neck, back and abdominal muscles, are particularly valuable for football players and wrestlers. They should be incorporated into the Advanced Level schedule. It is recommended you consult with your coach before adding them to your program.

Schedule

		Repetitions	
Page No.	Exercise	Minimum	Maximum
27	Rocking Chair	5	10
27	Wrestler's Bridge	5	10
28	Leg Lift with Chin Curl	5	10
29	Prone Raise	5	10

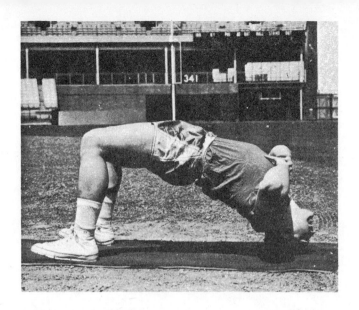

Wrestler's Bridge: Stretch out on your back with arms straight out to the side and knees bent so that feet are flat on the ground. Raise your body in an arch, with your weight resting on your feet and head. Use your arms only to keep your balance. Return to starting position.

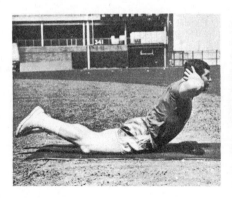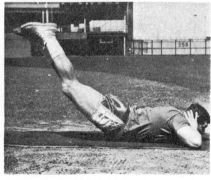

Rocking Chair: Lie on the floor on your stomach with hands clasped behind your head and with your legs together. Raise chest and legs and rock back and forth on stomach. Keep head up and legs as high as you can. Return to starting position.

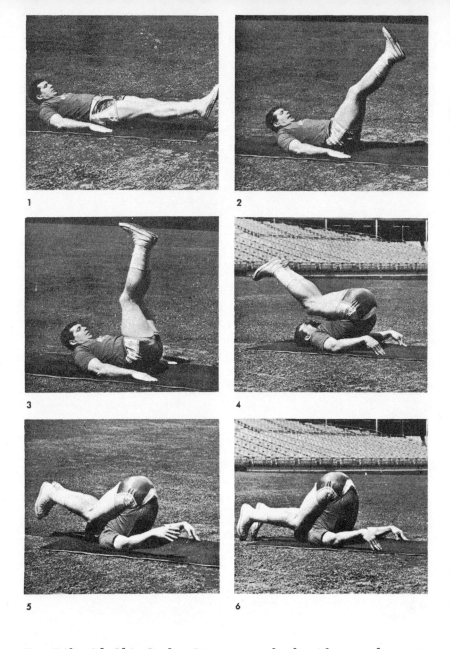

1   2
3   4
5   6

Leg Lift with Chin Curl: Lie on your back with arms down at your side and legs straight and together. Raise your legs and bring them over until your toes are touching the floor by your head. Hold for a second and return to starting position.

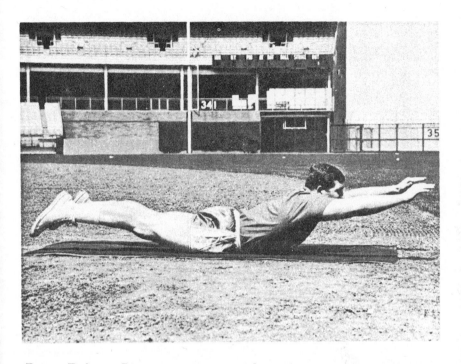

Prone Raise: Lie on your stomach with arms outstretched, fingers forward and thumbs touching. Legs should be straight and together. In same motion, raise arms and legs off floor, keeping them as straight as possible. Hold for a second and return to starting position.

Note: The daily workout may be skipped on any day in which you compete in a sport, provided it is reasonably strenuous.

5

Isometric Exercises

It is advisable not to start isometric exercises unless you have already worked your way into fairly good over-all condition. The purpose of doing isometrics is to *strengthen* muscles. This is accomplished by pushing, pulling or lifting against an immovable object or another resisting force.

The widespread enthusiasm for isometrics in recent years has given rise to the notion that they are complete conditioners in themselves. Not so. Since isometrics involve muscular contraction, they do not provide the necessary movement and flexibility for the muscles obtained by calisthenics and stretching exercises. Isometrics also do not greatly increase muscle size or endurance. They should not replace calisthenics in your conditioning program, but rather should serve as a valuable addition, according to your goals, since isometrics are excellent strength-builders.

The principle of isometrics is to maintain maximum tension on the muscle for several seconds. However, you should work up to that point slowly. At first, exert less than a maximum force and gradually increase your effort until you are at the maximum for the full six-second period. It will normally take about two weeks to build to a maximum muscle contraction and another two to three weeks before a noticeable gain in strength is apparent.

Do not hold your breath during an exercise. Take a deep breath at the start of the exercise and then exhale slowly.

One advantage of isometric exercises is that you do not have to perform the complete set to derive benefits from them. You can be selective and choose those exercises for the muscles you want to build up and concentrate on them. Another advantage is that isometrics, unlike weight-lifting, can be done every day. Also, they do not require special equipment.

Since the muscle will grow stronger primarily at the angle at which the isometric is performed, it is best to change the angle on the second and third repetitions whenever possible.

As with any exercise, you should modify an isometric exercise if pain results.

FOR THE LEGS

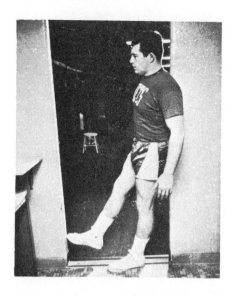

No. 1. Stand facing door jamb. Place right forefoot against door frame, keeping leg straight. Push forward and hold for six seconds. Repeat for left foot and hold for six seconds. Exercise each leg three times.

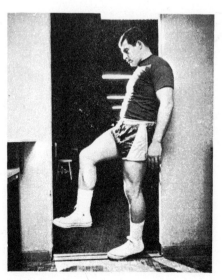

No. 2. Same exercise but with leg bent.

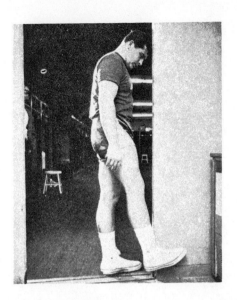

No. 3. Face door jamb. Step to left and hook right forefoot against the right side of door frame, keeping leg straight. Force right foot to left for six seconds. Repeat for left foot. Do each exercise three times.

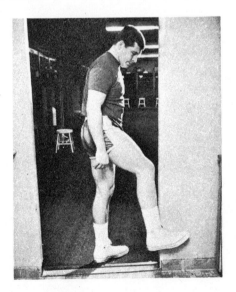

No. 4. Same exercise but with knee bent.

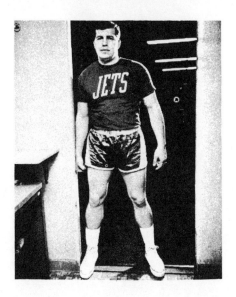

No. 1. Stand against door jamb. Place toes of right foot against opposite door jamb, keeping leg straight. Press toes forward and hold for six seconds. Repeat for left foot. Do each exercise three times.

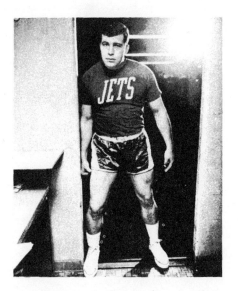

No. 2. Same exercise but with knee bent.

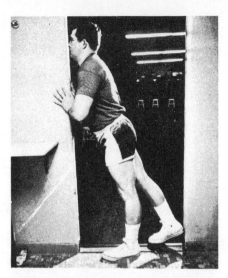

No. 3. Face door jamb and hold frame. Place right heel backward against opposite door jamb, keeping leg straight. Press heel against door jamb and hold for six seconds. Repeat with left heel. Do each exercise three times.

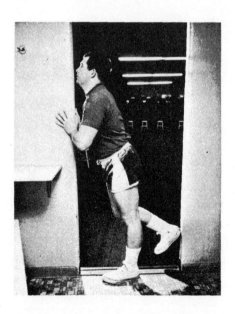

No. 4. Same exercise but with leg bent.

FOR THE ARMS

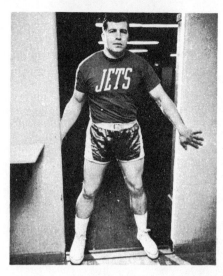

No. 1. Stand in doorway with arms at side. Grasp right door jamb with right hand, palm facing forward. Grasp left door jamb with left hand, palm facing backward. Push forward with right hand and backward with left hand for six seconds. Reverse hand positions and repeat. Do each exercise three times.

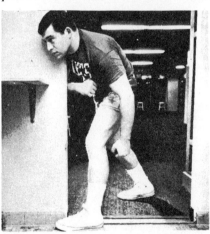

No. 2. Bend the knees and crouch, somewhat similar to blocking stance in football. Place left foot against left side of door frame. Keep head on left side and pinch frame between head and right shoulder. Hold for six seconds and repeat on opposite side.

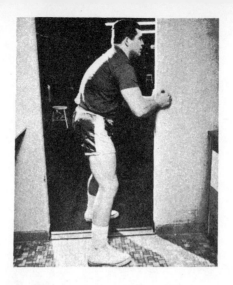

No. 3. Flex at hips, knees and ankles, with elbows wide. Place right hand around door frame and left hand on opposite side of door frame. Pull with right hand and push with left for six seconds. Repeat with left hand. Do each exercise three times.

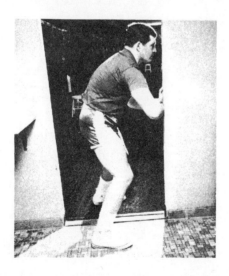

No. 4. Flex at hips, knees and ankles. Hold door frame with left hand and place at hip height against door frame. Press forward for six seconds. Reverse hands. Do each exercise three times.

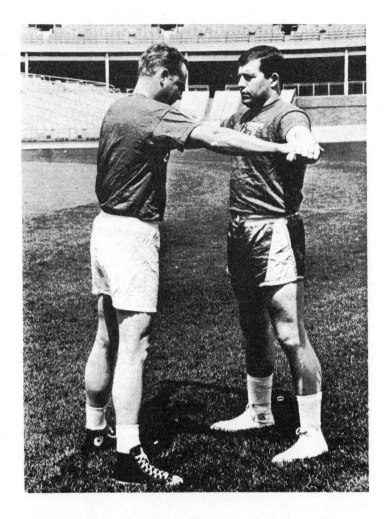

No. 1. A and B stand facing each other about 18 inches apart. A raises his arms to the side until they are level with his shoulders. B grasps A's arms just above the wrist.

A attempts to bring his arms together while B resists. Hold for six to eight seconds. Repeat after a 10-second rest. So that the muscles may be worked at different angles, A should bring his arms slightly closer together and repeat the exercise. Repeat a third time with A's arms again closer together.

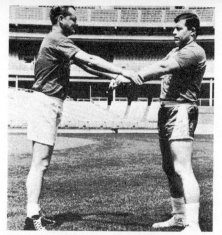

No. 2. A and B stand facing each other about 18 inches apart. A's arms should be straight and about 30 degrees forward. B grasps A's arms just above the wrist.

A pushes forward and upward while B resists. A should not bend his arms and should lift from the shoulders. Hold for six to eight seconds. Repeat twice, shortening the angle each time.

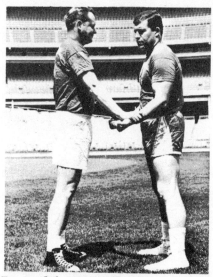

No. 3. A and B stand facing each other about 18 inches apart. A stands with arms parallel and elbows bent as if he were curling a weight. The angle of pull should be greater than a right angle. B grasps A's arms just above the wrists.

A attempts to flex his arms while B resists. Hold for six to eight seconds. Repeat twice, closing the angle to 90 degrees and then less than 90 degrees.

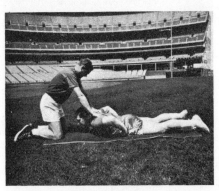

No. 4. A is in prone position (on stomach) with hands clasped on hips. B kneels at A's head with hands on A's shoulders.

A attempts to lift head and shoulders off the ground while B resists. Hold for six to eight seconds. Do the exercise three times.

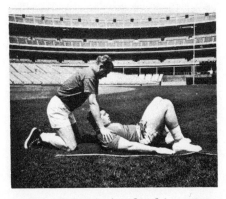

No. 5. A is in supine position (on back) with arms at side and palms down. A's feet should be drawn up with feet flat. B kneels at A's head with hands on A's shoulders.

A attempts to do a sit-up while B resists. Hold for six to eight seconds. Do the exercise three times. (NOTE: B should be careful not to apply too great resistance.)

Caution: Do not use isometrics to rebuild muscles after an injury or operation.

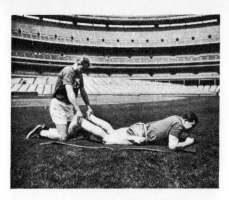

No. 6. A is in prone position on elbows. B kneels at A's feet and grasps A's heels.

A attempts to flex lower legs while B resists. Hold for six to eight seconds. Repeat twice, decreasing the angle the second time.

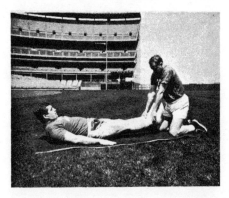

No. 7. A is in supine position (on back) with arms at side and palms down. B kneels at A's feet and grasps A just above the ankles.

Keeping legs straight, A attempts to do a straight leg lift while B resists. Hold for six to eight seconds. Repeat twice, decreasing the angle the second time.

6

Weight-Lifting

Weight-lifting is recommended primarily for the serious athlete who wants to build up his body as well as his strength. In the past, there had been misgivings in some quarters about the usefulness of weight-lifting in a sound conditioning program. It was feared that lifting weights might make an athlete "muscle-bound" and slow his coordination and muscular reactions. Those fears have been found to be groundless as long as the athlete continues to do calisthenics and guards against handling weights that are too heavy.

Weight-lifting is superior to isometrics as a body-builder because the movement involved increases muscular size and endurance in addition to strength.

Since it is strenuous exercise, weight-lifting should not be done on a daily basis but on alternate days.

Before each workout a warm-up is essential to prepare the muscles. Performing a few calisthenics, such as jumping jacks, arm circles, side twisters and running in place, for several minutes will suffice.

Another warm-up routine is to pick a weight well within your ability to handle in any exercise. Bend from the hips and grasp the bar with palms facing you, with the hands shoulder-width apart. Lift the weight, keeping your back straight. Then lean backwards with the weight hanging across the thighs. Repeat three to five times. Then pull the weight to the chest and repeat three to five times. Complete the warm-up by pulling the weight to the chest and then pushing it over the head three to five times.

The suggested starting weight for each exercise is considered to be a minimum one, but if you find the weight too heavy to perform the exercise comfortably, take a five-pound plate, or more if necessary, off the barbell. Always be sure to take a three-minute rest between sets.

If you find the suggested starting weights too light, increase the weight by five pounds. A good rule to follow, as you grow stronger, is to raise the number of repetitions first, then the number of sets before adding more weights. However, it may be four weeks before you notice any improvement in your physical condition.

Caution: If you have had an injury or an operation, consult your doctor for his approval of your weight-lifting program.

Weight-Lifting Schedule

(After calisthenics or light weight-lifting as warm-up exercise. Take three-minute rest between sets.)

Page No.	Exercise	Weight	Repetitions	Sets
43	Military Press	50 lbs.	5	2
44	Curl	30 lbs.	5	2
45	Side Twister	50 lbs.	5	2
46	Dead Lift	50 lbs.	5	2
46	Shoulder Shrug	50 lbs.	5	2
47	Bench Press	60 lbs.	5	2
48	Upright Rowing	50 lbs.	5	2
49	Bent Over Rowing	50 lbs.	5	2
50	Half Squats	50 lbs.	5	2

Until you become very expert at handling them, it is preferable not to work with the weights alone. A friend standing by can be helpful if the weight being lifted is too heavy, or if some other difficulty arises. This is especially true for the bench press exercise, which can be dangerous.

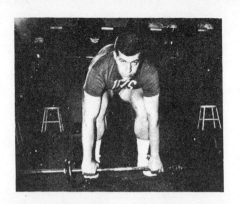

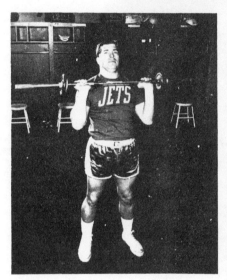

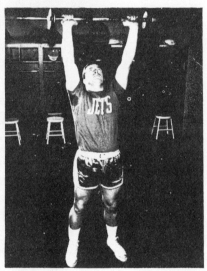

Military Press: In the starting position, stand with feet shoulder-width apart. Bend knees and grasp barbell with palms toward the floor and hands about shoulder-width apart. Raise weight to chest and hold so that palms face outward; the legs should be straight. Then push weight up until the arms are fully extended over the head. Important: Your eyes should be on the weight. Body should be erect. Do not use the legs to help get the weight up. Lower weight to chest and then raise weight again. Inhale as the weight is raised and exhale as weight is lowered. Develops: Upper arms, shoulders and neck. Goal: Lifting one-half your body weight.

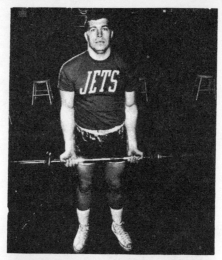

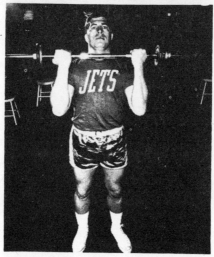

Curl: Grasp the barbell with the palms away from the legs and raise the weights to a hang position across the thighs. The handhold should be approximately shoulder-width apart and the arms should be extended with the elbows locked. Stand erect. Raise the weight to the chest by flexing the arms; lower weight to the starting position and repeat. Keep the elbows tucked at the sides. Keep your back straight and do not sway to help raise the bar. Stand with your back resting on a wall to prevent any swaying motion. Inhale as the bar is raised to the chest, exhale as it is lowered to the thighs. Develops: Biceps and forearm muscles. Goal: Lifting one-third your body weight.

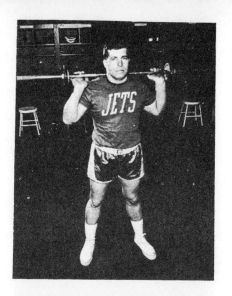

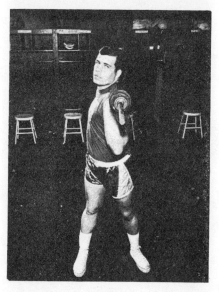

Side Twister: Place the barbell across the shoulders at the back of the neck with feet apart. The hands should be spaced slightly more than shoulder-width apart. Twist your trunk to the left as far as possible. Keep feet straight and head up. Return to starting position, then twist to your right as far as possible and return. Develops: Abdominal muscles. Goal: Lifting one-fourth your body weight.

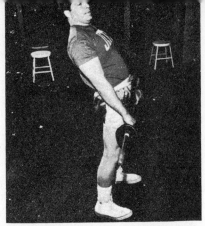

Dead Lift: Set feet about shoulder-width apart and grasp barbell with one palm toward the body and the other palm away. Knees should be flexed before starting to raise weight in order to put proper resistance on leg muscles. Lift bar until you are in a standing position, with knees straight and shoulders back. Lower weight until it is three or four inches from floor and then raise again to the erect position. Develops: Lower back muscles. Goal: Lifting one-third your body weight.

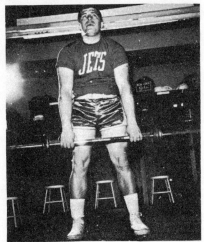

Shoulder Shrugs (can be combined with Dead Lift): After weight is raised to erect position, shrug the shoulders in a clockwise rotation for the five repetitions and then shrug the shoulders in a counterclockwise rotation for the five repetitions. Inhale as you shrug the shoulders and exhale as you relax the shoulders. Develops: Shoulder muscles. Goal: Lifting one-third to one-half your body weight.

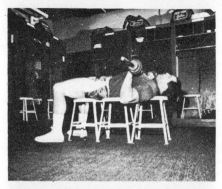

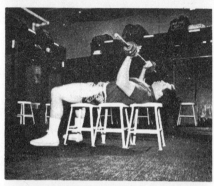

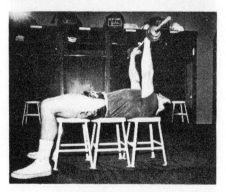

Bench Press: Lie flat on your back on a bench. The feet should be flat on the floor. The weight rests on your chest. Grasp the barbell with your hands about shoulder-width apart. Push the barbell straight up to arm's length with the elbows locked. Lower barbell to starting position and repeat. Inhale as you raise barbell and exhale as you lower barbell. Develops: Upper body, shoulders, chest, forearms and wrists. Goal: Lifting one-third to three-fifths your body weight.

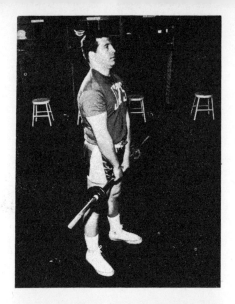

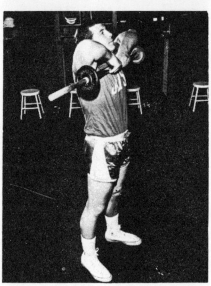

Upright Rowing: Grasp barbell with palms toward the floor. Hands should be about nine to 12 inches apart. Raise weight to hang position (across thighs.) Keep legs and body straight. Pull the weight straight up to the chin. Lower to hang position and repeat. Develops: Shoulders, upper arm and upper back muscles. Goal: Lifting one-quarter to one-half your body weight.

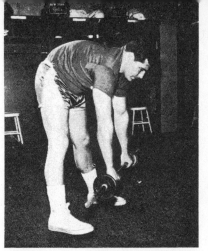

1

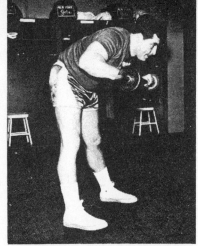

2

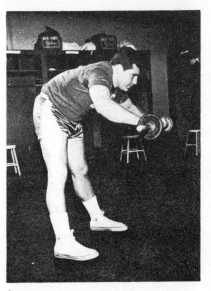

3

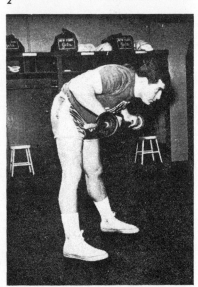

4

Bent Over Rowing: Grasp barbell with palms toward floor and hands about shoulder-width apart. Feet should be farther apart than shoulder-width. Back should be parallel to floor and legs should be straight. Raise weight to chest and then push weight forward and down and back in circular motion, simulating a rower's movement. Be sure to keep head up. Do not use body or leg motion to help bring the weight up. Inhale as you pull the weight up and exhale as you lower the weight. Develops: Upper back and arms. Goal: Lifting one-quarter to one-half your body weight.

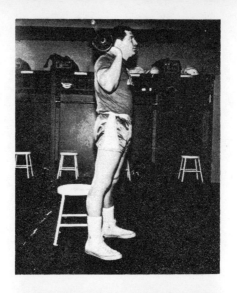

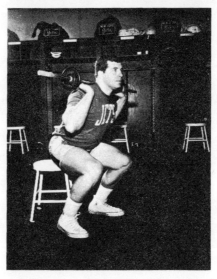

Half-Squat: Place barbell across the shoulders at the back of the neck. Feet are about shoulder-width apart, with toes pointing slightly outward. Keep back straight and bend down to a half-squat. Use a bench or stool to stop you from going into a full squat, but do not sit down. Head should be kept up. Raise your heels to maintain proper balance. Return to erect position and repeat. Develops: Thigh and leg muscles. Goal: Lifting three-quarters of body weight.

7

Stretching and Strengthening Exercises

A remarkable phenomenon has occurred in the New York Jets' training camp in recent years: No player has suffered a serious muscle strain or "pull"! This is an impressive record, as any coach on a high school, college or professional level can attest.

A "pull" (tear in the muscle) is about the most common injury players will sustain as they work to get into peak form for the season ahead. Such an injury will sideline a player for several days or for even as long as two or three weeks. Not only is his physical progress held back, but he also misses out on running through plays, scrimmaging and all the other preparations so vital to his career and the team's welfare.

The explanation for the Jets' success in this area is attributable to the theory and exercises developed by Dr. James Nicholas, the team physician and an orthopedic surgeon. Every player undergoes an examination by Dr. Nicholas. Through tests he has devised, Dr. Nicholas is able to determine whether an athlete may have some "tight" or "loose" muscles. Tight muscles, which tend to be stronger and more durable, are also the ones that are susceptible to "pulls." Loose muscles, which provide more agility, often need strengthening exercises, which are shown in the next section.

For tight muscles the recommended treatment is stretching exercises to make them more flexible. The following are some that have proved so beneficial to the Jets' players.

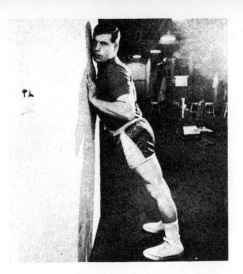

FOR THE CALF

Face a wall, at a distance of 12 to 15 inches, and place your hands on the wall a few inches below shoulder level. Making sure that your heels stay on the ground, move your body forward until your face reaches the wall. At this point the heels will be down, the knees back and the chest against the wall. There should be a slight pull felt in the calf muscles. Push away from the wall and repeat this exercise 10 times. This should be done in the morning and at night until the pull in the legs disappears. As you become more limber, you should move away from the wall to about 15 to 18 inches.

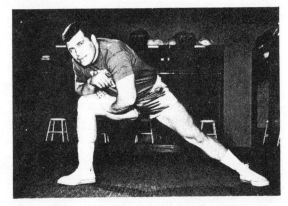

FOR THE GROIN

Take a long step with the right foot. Bend forward and try to touch your chest to the knee. Return to original position and then step forward with your left foot and try to touch your chest to the bent knee. Repeat with each leg four times.

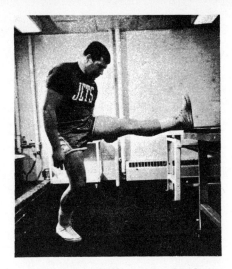

FOR THE THIGH

Stand and place the heel on a table or a desk, with the knee straight. Bend the opposite knee until the leg on the table is parallel to the floor. Repeat this five times on each leg until the pull in the thigh disappears. Be sure to keep the foot pointed toward your face.

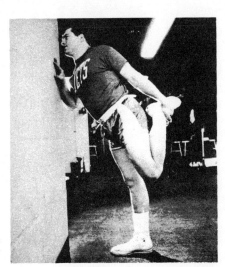

FOR THE FRONT THIGH

Stand with one hand resting on the wall. Grasp the opposite ankle and bring it to the buttock, as far back as possible, until either the heel touches the buttock or until you feel a tightness in the thigh. Repeat five times until the pull disappears. Do not bend forward if possible.

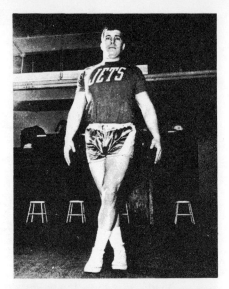

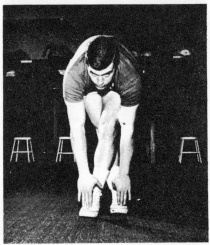

FOR THE HAMSTRING MUSCLE

In a standing position, cross your left foot over your right. Bend down and attempt to touch your toes keeping the knees straight. Then cross your right foot over your left and try to touch your toes again. Repeat each way four times.

Do not force or strain to touch toes since it is possible to be fit without the ability to touch your toes. It is suggested that more time be spent with thigh-stretching exercise (page 53) if you have difficulty with this exercise.

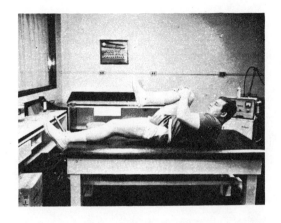

Lie flat on your back on a table or on the floor. Bend the right knee and bring it parallel to the chest at the level of your breast, keeping the left leg on the floor with the left knee completely straight. This should be done five consecutive times with each leg.

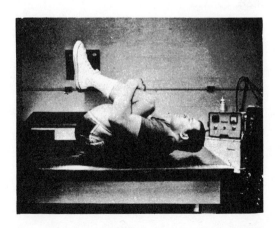

The same exercise, but do it with both legs together. The knees should come up against the chest. Repeat five times.

STRENGTHENING EXERCISES

To strengthen muscles in the leg, whether the result of being "loose" or previous injury or surgery, here are some of the exercises used by Jets' players:

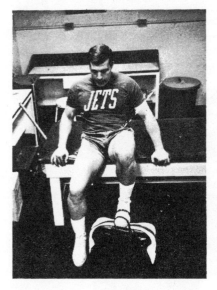 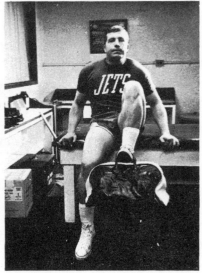

1. Fill a small canvas bag, such as an overnight, airline or traveling bag, with weights or books of about 20 to 25 pounds. Sit over a high desk or table with the knees bent. Hook the bag over one foot. Determine what the maximum weight is that one leg can lift and record it. Do the same for the opposite leg. Note the difference between the stronger and weaker leg so that you know what goal to aim for.

Hook the bag on the weaker leg. In the sitting position, with the leg bent at right angles, lift the leg 25 times to about the level of the breast, holding it for a second. The weight lifted should not be so heavy that you cannot complete the exercise without discomfort. It should not produce a cramp or a pull in the groin or cause breathlessness.

After four or five days, add a pound or two depending on how much the leg can carry. As a guideline, an athlete with strong thighs should be able to lift about 8 to 12 per cent of his body weight 25 times.

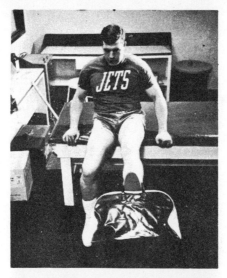

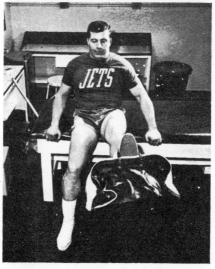

2. The same exercise except that you lift the weight with your leg held straight. Repeat 10 times.

WATER WALKING

An excellent summer exercise, to develop the thighs. In water up to the level of the groin, walk about 100 yards, keeping the knees stiff.

8

For the Weekend Sportsman
(Age 25 or over)

Your school days are in back of you and, most probably, so are organized team sports. For recreation perhaps you're a bowler, golfer, tennis player or an outdoorsman. In that respect you're ahead of your friends whose idea of taking part in a sport is to root for their favorite team from the stands or by the television set. But don't be misled that the weekly 18 holes of golf or the occasional trek into the woods is all you need to keep physically fit. You still require a consistent and balanced program of exercises to tone up all the muscles. Another "plus" of regular exercise is that it also is likely to improve your sports performance by lessening fatigue and increasing endurance and stamina.

As a sports "weekender" you have to be careful to avoid one risk. After five days of relative inactivity you can't afford to "go all out" and overextend yourself unless you're in very good condition. The Physical Fitness Test on page 6 will tell you what kind of shape you're in.

For those of you well over 25, another check on your general condition is to compare your present weight with what it was at 25. If the difference is more than 15 pounds, you should consult your doctor about going on a diet as well as a conditioning program.

Because of the many variable factors such as age, body build and athletic history, you should modify the following exercises to suit your particular requirements. Try to maintain a Monday-through-Friday schedule on the calisthenics and perform them at about the same time each day so that they become a normal part of your routine.

STRETCHING EXERCISES

As you get older, you tend to lose flexibility and suppleness of muscle. If you suffer from spasms or cramps in the calves, do the exercise on page 52. To make the back muscles more limber, do the exercise on page 55.

CALISTHENICS

Page No.	Exercise	Starting Repetitions
10	Jumping Jacks	10
9	Arm Circles (each way)	20
11	Side Twisters	10
13	Sit-Ups	5
19	Knee to Chest (each knee)	5
14	Push-Ups	5
15	Running in Place	100 counts

Increase repetitions by five each if starting program proves too easy, and continue to increase until total repetitions are triple the basic number. For more variety, add toe touching (page 12), on all four's (page 17) and leg crossover (page 18) to schedule desired.

For those in non-running sports, such as *bowling, golf* and *skiing*: Run-Walk exercise is recommended three times a week to build wind endurance and make up for lack of running in sport.

Run at a slow pace—at a jog or trot—until you become winded. Then walk until you recover and resume running. Start with distance of half-mile and increase gradually.

Whenever an exercise proves difficult, reduce the number of repetitions until you have mastered it.

ISOMETRICS

For **tennis, handball** and **skiing:** Strengthen leg muscles by adding exercises on pages 31-34.

For **golf:** Strengthen arm and shoulder muscles by adding exercises on pages 35-36.

WEIGHT-LIFTING

Unless you've had previous experience with weights, it's not recommended you add it to your conditioning program. For those who know how to lift weights, a moderate schedule is suggested. Be sure the weight you handle is easily within your ability. It is preferable to increase repetitions rather than putting more plates on the barbell.

For the upper arms, shoulders and wrists, try the military press on page 43, the shoulder shrug on page 46, and upright rowing on page 48.

The hazards of cigarette smoking have been well publicized. As an adult this is your decision to make. If you can't or won't give up smoking, minimize the harmful effects by smoking 10 or less cigarettes each day. Avoid smoking a cigarette immediately before exercising vigorously.

9

Exercises for Girls

Perhaps you never thought of exercising as a beauty aid. You should. Regular exercise can enhance your appearance, for example, in such ways as helping to give you better posture, to keep your body trim and even to improve your complexion! In addition, your normal growth and development depend on strengthening your muscles, heart and lungs so that they can do their jobs well. When you are physically fit, you discover that you are better able to do the things you want to do and you have more fun doing them. Don't think that only girls with athletic ambitions should exercise regularly.

The calisthenics program that has been prepared is intended to supplement whatever exercising you may do at school. Try to make doing the calisthenics a regular habit. It will also be helpful if you can exercise at about the same time each day.

Read the descriptions under the photographs carefully, since it is important to do each exercise properly. Be more concerned with performing each exercise thoroughly rather than with speed. You are not competing with anyone else—only with yourself.

Rest during the exercises whenever you become too winded or fatigued. Doing exercises until they "hurt" is wrong. If you have passed a medical examination recently—and you should have one at least once a year—the chances are that you will be able to complete the minimum schedule on the Basic Level without too much trouble and, in a short time, to do the exercises without taking "breathers."

Increase the repetitions to the maximum number as the exercises become easier to do. Don't go on to the Advanced Level until you are able to complete the maximum schedule comfortably on a daily basis for two weeks.

Basic Level Schedule*

Page No.	Exercise	Repetitions	
		Minimum	Maximum
63	Jumping Jacks	5	10
64	Head Bobs	4	8
64	Wing Stretchers	4	8
65	Arm Circles (each way)	10	20
65	Stretch and Toe Touch	6	10
66	Waist Bobs (each way)	4	8
67	Front Straddle, Head to Knee (each side)	4	8
67	Leg Raisers (each side)	4	8
68	Sit-Ups **	10	15
69	Running in place	50 counts	

* The daily workout may be skipped on any day in which you engage in a vigorous athletic activity, such as swimming or playing tennis.

** If you can't bend over and touch toes at first, touch knees until you become able to complete the exercise.

Whenever an exercise proves difficult, reduce the number of repetitions until you have mastered it.

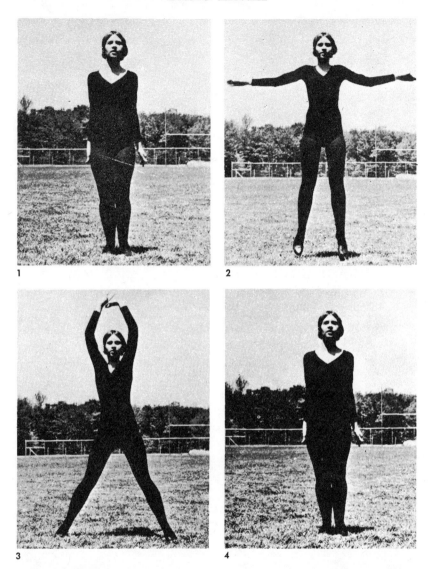

Jumping Jacks: Assume an at-attention position, with shoulders back, chest out, stomach in and arms straight down. Swing your arms in a full arc over your head until your fingers touch and simultaneously jump so that your feet land about shoulder-width apart. Hold for an instant and jump back to starting position. Hold for an instant and repeat. The exercise should be done in an almost continuous, rhythmic motion.

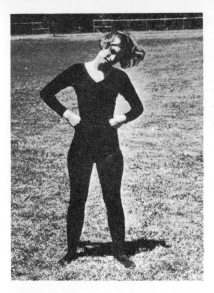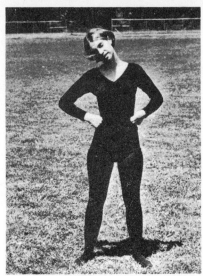

Head Bobs: Start with hands on hips, keeping back straight and moving head and neck only. Bob the head back four times, then to the left four times, then to the right four times and then forward four times.

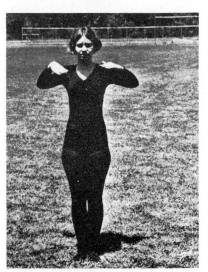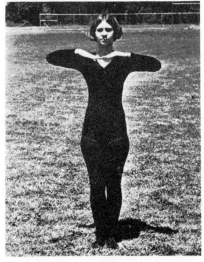

Wing Stretchers: Place arms at chest-height with elbows bent and fingertips touching. Using shoulder muscles, pull elbows back as far as you can, return and repeat, keeping the arms up. Then swing the arms straight out to the side, return and repeat.

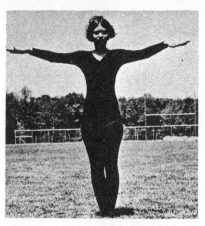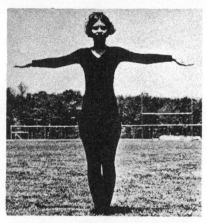

Arm Circles: Extend arms directly out to the side at shoulder height with palms down, fingers straight and together. Rotate the shoulders in forward motion so that the arms describe circles of about a foot in diameter. At the same time arch the head backward and turn it slowly to the left and to the right. After completing the specified number of repetitions, rotate the shoulders in a backward motion for the same number of repetitions. Be sure to keep the arms straight and do not let them "droop."

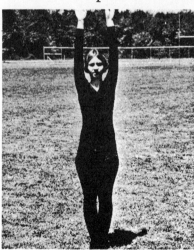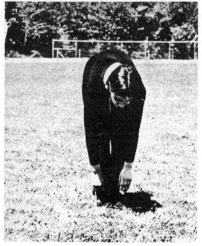

Stretch and Toe Touch: From at-attention position, extend arms upward over head on count one. Bend over and try to touch toes—or as close as you can—on count two. Straighten up and place hands on hips on count three. Return to starting position on count four. In trying to touch toes, do not force. Avoid strain to lower back and calves.

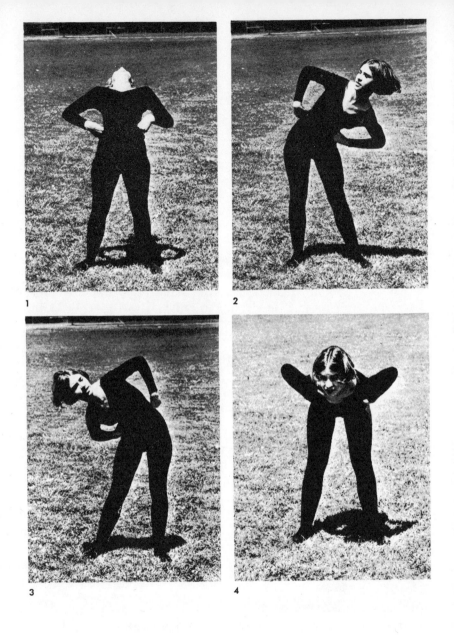

Waist Bobs: Place hands on hips, legs shoulder-width apart with knees straight. Bob from the waist backward four times, then to the left four times, then to the right four times, then forward four times.

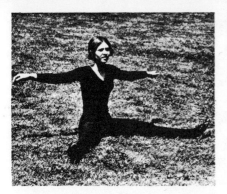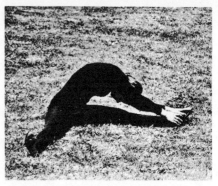

Front Straddle, Head to Knee: Sit erect with legs apart and hands on hips. Bend to the left, trying to touch head to left knee and hands to toes. Return to starting position and repeat to the right. You may have difficulty touching head to knee but you will achieve greater suppleness with practice.

Concentrate on those exercises that prove hardest to do properly with the required number of repetitions.

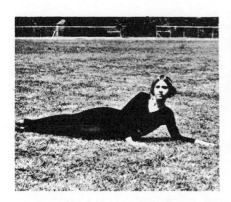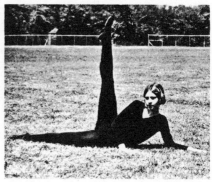

Leg Raisers: Lie on left side with legs straight and together and weight resting on left elbow. Swing right leg up as high as you can. Do not bend leg and do not slouch on your left side. Return to starting position. After the specified number of repetitions, turn over to your right side and repeat.

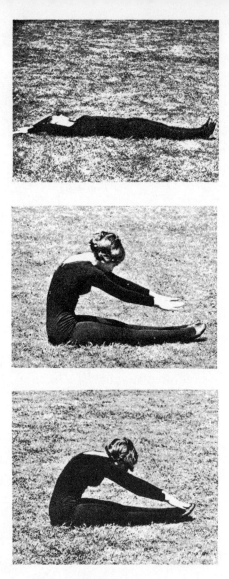

Sit-Ups: Stretch out on your back with arms over your head and legs together. Contracting stomach muscles, bring body up and try to touch toes. Return to starting position. If you have difficulty raising yourself, put your feet under a heavy object—such as a sofa or chair—to anchor them. Don't be concerned if you can't touch your toes at first. The important thing is to reach an upright position.

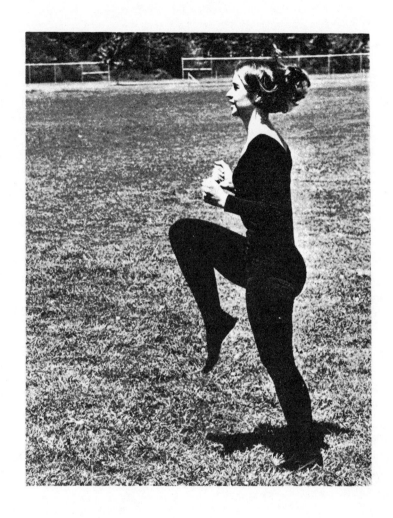

Running in place: Assume runner's position with elbows bent. Keep shoulders back and body straight. Lift legs at least six inches off floor. Count each time left foot hits floor. Start slowly and then speed up.

Advanced Level Schedule

| | | Repetitions | |
| | | Mini- | Maxi- |
Page No.	Exercise	mum	mum
63	Jumping Jacks	10	20
64	Head Bobs	8	10
64	Wing Stretchers	8	10
65	Arm Circles (each way)	20	30
65	Stretch and Toe Touch	10	15
66	Waist Bobs (each way)	10	15
67	Front Straddle, Head to Knee (each side)	8	12
71	Front Straddle, Elbows to Floor	8	12
72	Sprinter's Start	10	20
67	Leg Raisers (each side)	8	12
73	Leg Crossovers (each side)	6	12
68	Sit-Ups	20	30
69	Running in place	100 counts	

The daily workout may be skipped on any day in which you engage in a vigorous athletic activity, such as swimming or playing tennis.

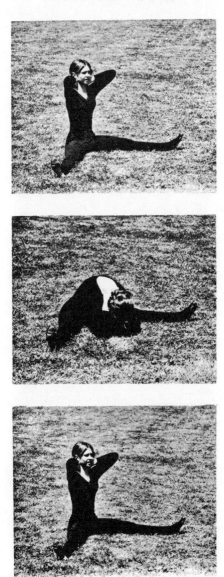

Front Straddle, Elbows to Floor: Sit erect with legs apart and hands clasped behind head. Bend forward and try to touch elbows to floor. Bob four times and then return to starting position.

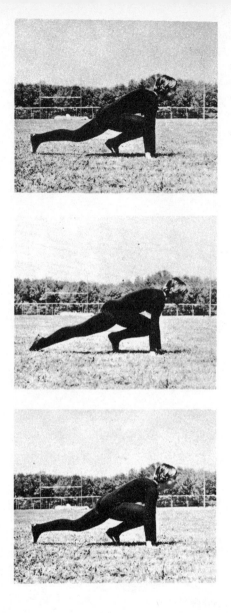

Sprinter's Start: Place hands on floor shoulder-width apart and extend right leg back and straight and left leg forward and bent. Switch leg positions and hold for a second. Return to starting position and repeat. Keep back up and elbows straight.

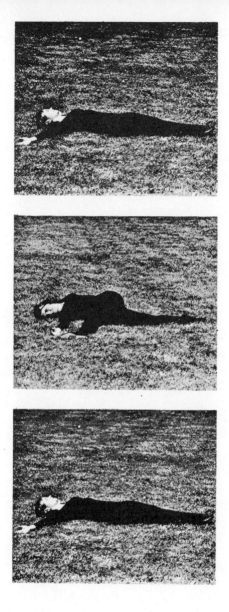

Leg Crossover: Stretch out with legs together and arms extended to the side. Lift right leg and cross over, twisting from the waist, and try to touch left hand with right foot. Return to starting position and repeat with other leg. Try to keep both legs straight.

10

Exercises for Women

If you're a busy housewife taking care of a family and a home, a conditioning program may sound like the last thing in the world you would need. But it is a fact that in your daily activities you tend to use the same muscles and you miss out on the benefits of an over-all conditioning program. This may be even more true if, instead, you are employed and your job is a sedentary one.

By undertaking a planned program of calisthenics, you tone up and firm all the major muscles and stimulate the circulatory system, enabling the heart and lungs to function more efficiently. In turn, this can lengthen life expectancy. Keeping fit can make you feel and look younger.

If you are overweight, exercising, by itself, will not help you lose the undesired pounds—what and how much you eat is the key factor here—but it will help to keep your weight down by burning up calories and providing you with an extra incentive to stay in condition.

It is best if you have a medical examination before starting your calisthenics program—you probably have one each year anyway—and your doctor may suggest some modifications in the exercises.

Try to exercise daily—and at the same time of the day if possible—so that it becomes a natural part of your routine.

Read the descriptions under the photographs carefully, since it is important to do each exercise properly. Be more concerned with performing all the exercises completely rather than with speed. You are not competing with anyone else—only with yourself.

To many, the minimum number of repetitions on the Basic Level may seem to be too easy. But do not be too hasty in going on to the maximum number. Be sure you can do all the exercises at the lower number comfortably without taking "breathers."

Rest whenever you become too winded or fatigued. For the first few days there may be a slight stiffness or soreness until your muscles become accustomed to the program, but there should not be any serious discomfort or pain.

Basic Level Schedule

| Page No. | Exercise | Repetitions | |
		Mini-mum	Maxi-mum
76	Jumping Jacks	5	10
77	Arm Circles (each way)	10	20
78	Side Twisters	6	12
79	Toe Raisers	5	10
80	Toe Touches	4	8
81	Sit-Ups *	8	12
82	Knee Push-Ups	6	10
83	Running in place	50 counts	

* This likely will prove to be the most difficult exercise. If you can't bend over and touch the toes at first, touch knees until you are able to complete the exercise.

When you are able to perform all the exercises with the maximum repetitions easily in five minutes for one week, progress to the Medium Level.

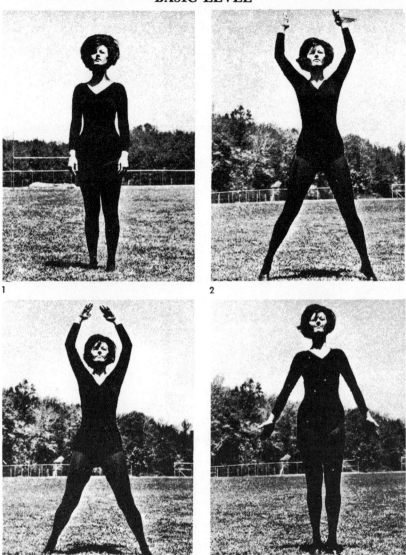

1

2

3

4

Jumping Jacks: Assume an at-attention position, with shoulders back, chest out, stomach in and arms straight down. Swing your arms in a full arc over your head until your fingers touch and simultaneously jump so that your feet land about shoulder-width apart. Hold for an instant and jump back to starting position. Hold for an instant and repeat. The exercise should be done in an almost continuous, rhythmic motion.

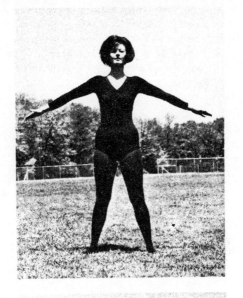

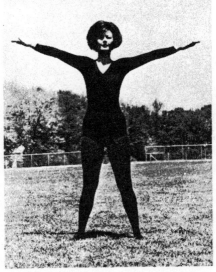

Arm Circles: Extend arms directly out to the side at shoulder height with palms down, fingers straight and together. Rotate the shoulders in forward motion so that the arms describe circles of about a foot in diameter. At the same time arch the head backward and turn it slowly to the left and to the right. After completing the specified number of repetitions, rotate the shoulders in a backward motion for the same number of repetitions. Be sure to keep the arms straight and do not let them "droop."

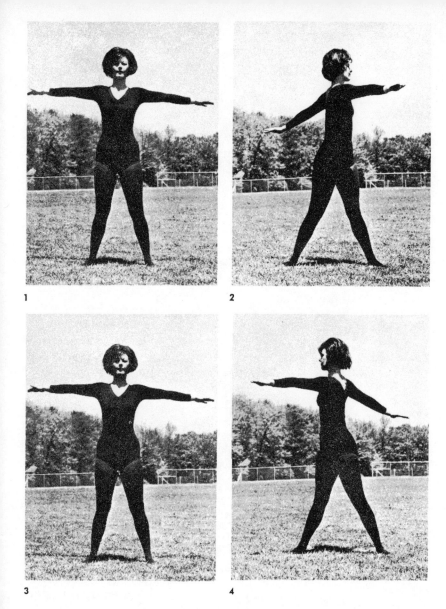

Side Twisters: Place feet shoulder-width apart and arms extended straight to the side at shoulder-level. Keeping feet stationary, twist trunk to the left as far as you can and return to starting position. Then twist to the right as far as you can and return. Keep arms straight and do not let them drop.

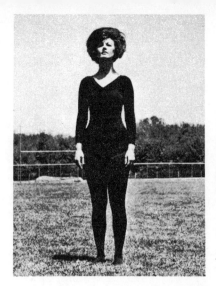
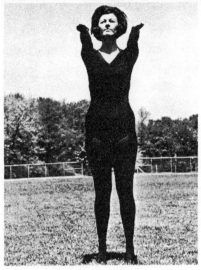
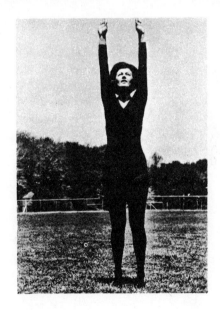

Toe Raisers: From at-attention position, slowly (to a count of four) raise up on your toes and simultaneously bring your arms straight up, reaching as high as you can. Hold for a second. Inhale through the mouth on your way up and exhale through your nose on the way down.

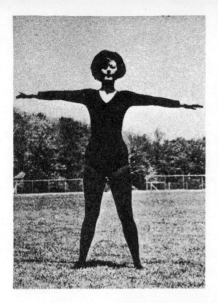
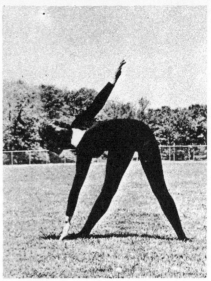
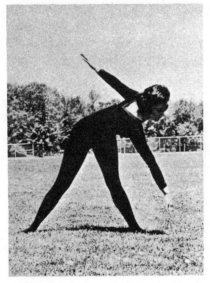

Toe Touches: Place feet shoulder-width apart and arms extended to the side at shoulder-level. Bending from waist, try to touch right foot—or as close as you can—with left hand, keeping knees straight. Return to starting position and repeat with right hand to left foot. Avoid strain to lower back and calves.

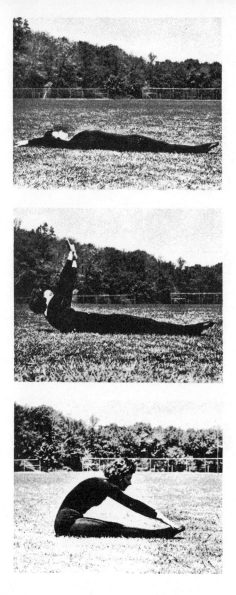

Sit-Ups: Stretch out on your back with arms over your head and legs together. Contracting stomach muscles, bring body up and try to touch toes. Return to starting position. If you have difficulty raising yourself, put your feet under a heavy object—such as a sofa or chair—to anchor them. Don't be concerned if you can't touch your toes at first. The important thing is to reach an upright position.

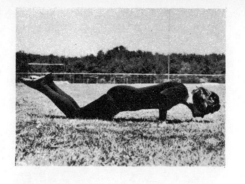

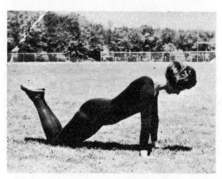

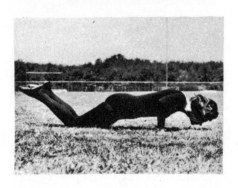

Knee Push-Ups: Stretch out on your stomach, with your hands underneath your shoulders, fingers forward. Push on your hands and raise yourself until your arms are straight and your body is resting on your hands and knees. Hold for a second and then lower your body until it nearly touches the floor. Then rise again. Keep your head up.

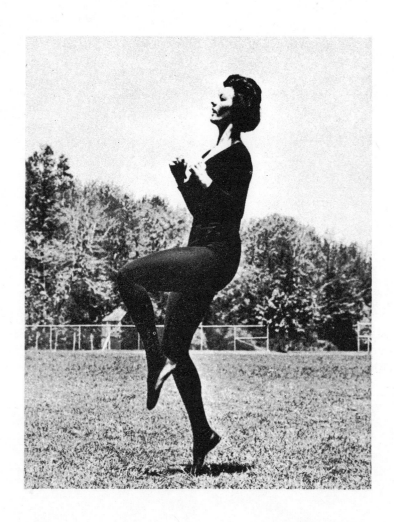

Running in place: Assume runner's position with elbows bent. Keep shoulders back and body straight. Lift legs at least six inches off floor. Count each time left foot hits floor. Start slowly and then speed up.

Medium Level Schedule

Page No.	Exercise	Repetitions Minimum	Maximum
76	Jumping Jacks	10	20
77	Arm Circles (each way)	20	30
78	Side Twisters	12	18
79	Toe Raisers	10	12
80	Toe Touches	8	12
84	Leg Raisers (each way)	6	12
85	Sprinter's Start	10	20
81	Sit-Ups	15	20
85	Regular Push-Ups	5	10
83	Running in place	100 counts	

How quickly you progress depends on many factors such as age, body build, general state of health and previous conditioning. For many it will be adequate to achieve the Medium Level with maximum number of repetitions in eight minutes.

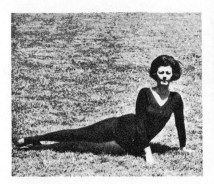 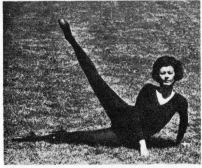

Leg Raisers: Lie on left side with legs straight and together and weight resting on left elbow. Swing right leg up as high as you can. Do not bend leg and do not slouch on your left side. Return to starting position. After the specified number of repetitions, turn over to your right side and repeat.

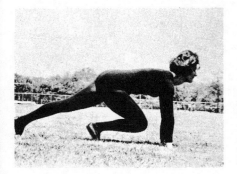 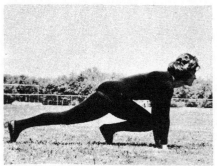

Sprinter's Start: Place hands on floor shoulder-width apart and extend right leg back and straight and left leg forward and bent. Switch leg positions and hold for a second. Return to starting position and repeat. Keep back up and elbows straight.

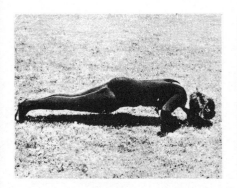 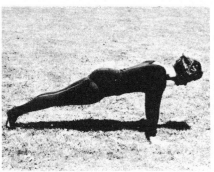

Regular Push-Ups: Stretch out on the floor on your stomach, with your hands underneath your shoulders, fingers forward. Push on your hands and raise yourself until your arms are straight and your body is resting on your hands and toes. Hold for a second and lower your body until it nearly touches the floor. Then raise yourself again. Don't let back sag—it should be straight—and don't push buttocks up first. The arms should do the work.

Advanced Level Schedule

Page No.	Exercise	Repetitions Mini-mum	Maxi-mum
76	Jumping Jacks	20	30
77	Arm Circles (each way)	30	40
78	Side Twisters	18	24
79	Toe Raisers	12	15
80	Toe Touches	12	15
84	Leg Raisers (each side)	12	18
87	Leg Crossovers	8	16
85	Sprinter's Start	20	30
87	Prone Raise	3	6
81	Sit-Ups	20	25
	or		
88	Abdominal Curls	6	10
85	Regular Push-Ups	10	15
83	Running in place	150 counts	

The daily workout may be skipped on any day in which you engage in a vigorous athletic activity, such as swimming or playing tennis.

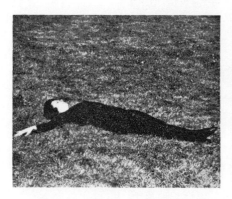 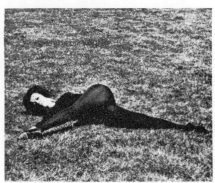

Leg Crossover: Stretch out with legs together and arms extended to the side. Lift right leg and cross over, twisting from the waist, and try to touch left hand with right foot. Return to starting position and repeat with other leg. Try to keep both legs straight.

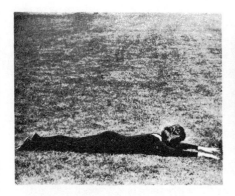 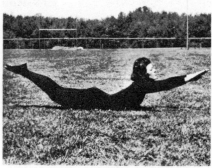

Prone Raise: Stretch out on your stomach with your arms extended straight ahead and your legs together. Raise arms and legs off floor as high as you can, keeping them straight. Return to starting position.

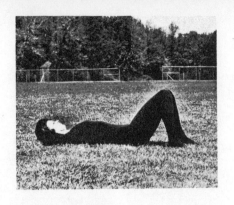

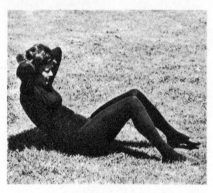

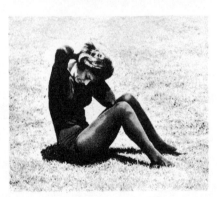

Abdominal Curl: Lie on your back with hands clasped behind head, knees bent and feet flat on the floor. Contracting stomach muscles, bring body up and touch elbows to knees and return to starting position. Try to keep feet flat on ground. Use the abdominal muscles and not the upper part of the body.

A "SPECIAL" FOR THE HOUSEWIFE

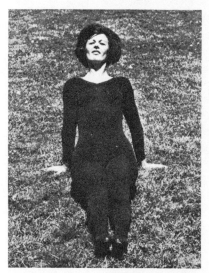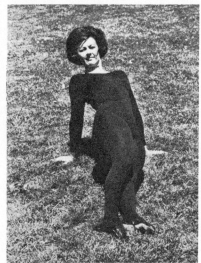

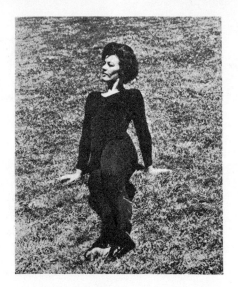

Hip Bouncer: Sit on floor with legs together and hands at sides. Raise hips off floor a few inches, with weight on hands and feet. In continuous movement, "thump" floor with hips eight times, then twist trunk to the left and "thump" floor with left hip eight times and twist to the right and "thump" floor eight times with right hip. Return to starting position. Repeat sequence with four "thumps" in each position, then two and then one in rapid tempo.

STRETCHING EXERCISES

Face a wall, at a distance of 12 to 15 inches, and place your hands on the wall a few inches below shoulder level. Making sure that your heels stay on the ground, move your body forward until your face reaches the wall. At this point the heels will be down, the knees back and the chest against the wall. There should be a slight pull felt in the calf muscles. Push away from the wall and repeat this exercise 10 times. This should be done in the morning and at night until the pull in the legs disappears. As you become more limber, you should move away from the wall to about 15 to 18 inches.

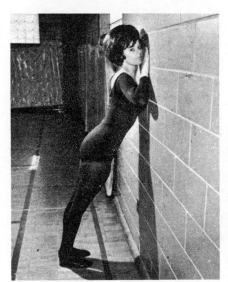

FOR THE CALF

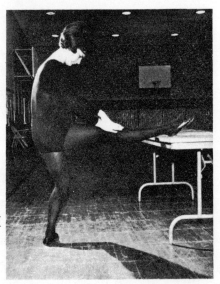

FOR THE THIGH

Stand and place the heel on a table or a desk, with the knee straight. Bend the opposite knee until the leg on the table is parallel to the floor. Repeat this five times on each leg until the pull in the thigh disappears. Be sure to keep the foot pointed toward your face.

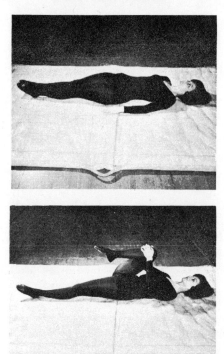

Lie flat on your back on a table or on the floor. Bend the right knee and bring it parallel to the chest at the level of your breast, keeping the left leg on the floor with the left knee completely straight. This should be done five consecutive times with each leg.

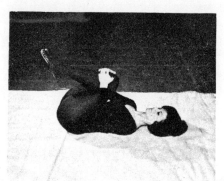

The same exercise, but do it with both legs together. The knees should come up against the chest. Repeat five times.

11

Diet

In this land of plenty, at least one of every four Americans is overweight, according to the American Medical Association. For this one-fourth of the population, the excess fat stored in the body places a greater strain on the heart and other internal organs and makes them more susceptible to high blood pressure, heart trouble and other disease.

By medical definition, you are considered to be overweight if you carry 10 per cent more weight than your normal weight.

The problem arises when more calories are consumed than the body burns up. An extra 100 calories a day, for example, can mean a gain of 10 pounds in a year. The total number of calories is not the key. An active person can have a daily intake of 3,500 calories and still not add weight, while 2,500 calories can be too many for a less active individual.

Pro football players are notoriously good eaters (some years ago, when the caliber of the teams was not as high as it is today, a coach described his squad as consisting of three fine players and 30 excellent eaters). In training camp the average player will get 4,000 calories and still not put on weight because he "works it off" in the practice sessions.

Some people are fortunate enough to keep their weight at a desired level with a few adjustments in their eating habits. Eliminating between-meal snacks is a frequent solution. Skipping high-calorie desserts or cutting down on the amount of sugar or butter often proves sufficient. Others continue to eat the same foods but take smaller portions. And regular exercises, of course, helps to burn up the extra calories.

Obviously, any severe dieting should be done only under a doctor's supervision.

In a balanced diet there should be daily servings of milk, cheese or other dairy products; meat, poultry, fish or eggs; fruits and vegetables, and breads and cereals. Excellent examples of nutritionally correct meals are the typical menus of the Jets that follow.

Monday	Tuesday

Breakfast

Chilled grapefruit juice
Chilled grapefruit-orange sections
Dry cereal
Eggs any style
Pork roll
Crisp hot toast
Butter
Peach preserves
Coffee—Milk

Lunch

Chilled apple juice
Old fashioned beef stew
Made with fresh vegetables
Buttered noodles
Potato chips
Chopped lettuce—Tomato
  wedges
Mayonnaise—Dressing
Chocolate fudge squares
Chocolate icing
Hot pan rolls—Butter
Iced Tea—Coffee

Dinner

Chicken rice soup
Saltines
Roast prime rib of beef
Creamy whipped potatoes
Buttered asparagus
Chef's tossed garden salad
French dressing
Cocoanut cream pie
Whipped cream rings
Toasted cocoanut
Muffin tin rolls—Butter
Iced Tea—Coffee—Milk

Breakfast

Chilled orange juice
Chilled Kadota figs
Dry cereal
Eggs any style
Grilled link sausage
Hot griddle cakes
Crisp hot toast
Butter
Syrup
Orange Marmalade
Coffee—Milk

Lunch

Chilled apricot nectar
Grilled jumbo hamburger
Sliced raw onions
Vegetable Chow—Chow
Hash—Brown potatoes
Mixed Garden Vegetables
Sliced Tomatoes—Lettuce
Mayonnaise—Dressing
Assorted Jello squares
Whipped Cream—Cookies
Hamburger Rolls—Butter
Iced Tea—Coffee

Dinner

Chilled melon balls
Roast leg of milk fed veal
Natural brown gravy
Celery dressing
Oven browned potatoes
Golden bantam corn
Chilled peach halves
Cottage cheese salad
Banana cream pie
Meringue topping
Parker House rolls—Butter
Iced Tea—Coffee—Milk

Wednesday	Thursday
Breakfast	*Breakfast*
Chilled orange-grapefruit juice	Chilled orange juice
Chilled cantaloupe	Chilled grapefruit sections
Dry cereal	Dry cereal
Eggs any style	Eggs any style
Rashers of bacon	Pork roll
Crisp hot toast	Crisp hot toast
Butter	Butter
Black cherry preserves	Strawberry preserves
Coffee—Milk	Coffee—Milk
Lunch	*Lunch*
Chilled grape juice	Chilled pineapple juice
Cold sliced roast beef	Boston style baked beans
Ham—Cheese	with diced frankfurters
Candied pickle sticks	Vegetable chow—Chow
Sweet relish	Sliced kosher pickles
Home style potato salad	Potato chips
Sliced Tomatoes—Lettuce	Shredded lettuce salad
Mayonnaise—Dressing	Italian dressing
Chilled sliced peaches	Rice Custard—with Raisins
Cookies	Vanilla sauce
Bread—Butter	Hot Dog Rolls—Butter
Iced Tea—Coffee	Iced Tea—Coffee
Dinner	*Dinner*
Old fashioned bean soup	Chilled fruit cocktail
Saltines	Yankee pot roast of beef
Grilled sirloin strip steak	Jardinere sauce
French fried potatoes	Creamy whipped potatoes
Fordhook lima beans	Blue lake green beans,
Head lettuce salad	Chef's sweet-sour salad
Blue cheese dressing	Sweet-sour vinegar dressing
Home made peach pie	Black and white layer cake
Rolls—Butter	Half and half icing
Iced Tea—Coffee—Milk	Crescent rolls—seeded
	Butter
	Iced Tea—Coffee—Milk

Friday	Saturday
Breakfast	*Breakfast*

Chilled grapefruit juice	Chilled orange-grapefruit juice
Sliced fresh peaches	Diced fresh oranges
Dry cereal	Dry cereal
Eggs any style	Eggs any style
Grilled link sausage	Rashers of bacon
Crisp hot toast	Crisp hot toast
Butter	Butter
Home made sticky buns	Cherry preserves
Blackberry preserves	Coffee—Milk
Coffee—Milk	

Lunch	*Lunch*
Chilled peach nectar	Chilled tomato juice
White meat albacore tuna salad	Saltines
Assorted cold cuts	Sautéed ground sirloin tips
Sweet cucumber slices	with tomato gravy
Mustard	Crisp hot toast
Home style macaroni salad	Sliced kosher pickles
Potato sticks	Potato chips
Sliced tomatoes—Lettuce	Pickle beet—Onion salad
Mayonnaise—Dressing	Sweet vinegar dressing
Chocolate cream dessert	Sliced pineapple rings
Whipped cream—Cookies	Cookies
Bread—Butter	Bread—Butter
Iced Tea—Coffee	Iced Tea—Coffee

Dinner	*Dinner*
Manhattan clam chowder	Chilled citrus salad
Saltines	Grilled sirloin strip steak
Jumbo butterfly shrimp	French fried potatoes
Baked Virginia cured ham	Buttered asparagus tips
Pineapple sauce—tartar sauce	Chef's combination salad
French fried potatoes	French dressing
Fresh frozen garden peas	Iced cold watermelon
Cole slaw salad	Bread—Butter
Boiled spiced dressing	Iced Tea—Coffee—Milk
Lemon meringue pie	
Meringue topping	
Parker House rolls	
Butter	
Iced Tea—Coffee—Milk	

Sunday

Breakfast

Chilled orange juice
Sliced bananas
Dry cereal
Eggs any style
Grilled link sausage
Hot griddle cakes
Crisp hot toast
Syrup
Pure apple jelly
Coffee—Milk

Lunch

Chilled fruit cocktail
Southern fried chicken
Supreme sauce
Creamy whipped potatoes
Buttered succotash
Celery hearts—Radishes
Stuffed queen olives
Home made cherry pie
Rolls
Butter
Iced Tea—Coffee

Dinner

Chicken noodle soup
Saltines
Assorted cold cuts
Candied pickle strips
Potato chips
Hot potato salad
Sliced tomatoes—Lettuce
Mayonnaise—Dressing
Ice cream sundae
Chocolate fudge sauce
Whole maraschino cherry
Bread—Butter
Iced Tea—Coffee
Milk